Robert Wasner
Alphonse Mancini

Slim through the syringe

A medical guide to weight loss injections

bup

Robert Wasner
Alphonse Mancini

Slim through the syringe

A medical guide to weight loss injections

ISBN: 978-3-68904-388-9 (Paperback)
ISBN: 978-3-68904-400-8 (e-book)

Copyright: Bremen University Press, Bremen, 2024. The manuscript may not be used in whole or in part without the prior written consent of the publisher.

First edition
Manuscript No. 1377
April 2024
Printed in the European Union
bup@bremenuniversitypress.com
www.bremenuniversitypress.com

Robert Wasner
Alphonse Mancini

Slim through the syringe

A medical guide to weight loss injections

Overview

INTRODUCTION TO THE TOPIC OF WEIGHT LOSS INJECTIONS	4
TYPES OF SLIMMING SYRINGES	10
THE SCIENCE BEHIND WEIGHT LOSS INJECTIONS	22
SUCCESS OF WEIGHT LOSS INJECTIONS	28
LONG-TERM EFFECTS AND SUSTAINABILITY OF WEIGHT LOSS	38
RISKS AND SIDE EFFECTS	41
WHICH SLIMMING INJECTION FOR WHOM?	63
OPTIMUM USE OF WEIGHT LOSS SYRINGES	83
SOURCES OF SUPPLY	92
ETHICAL AND SOCIAL CONSIDERATIONS	94
NEW DRUGS, CONCLUSION AND OUTLOOK	97

Table of contents

INTRODUCTION TO THE TOPIC OF WEIGHT LOSS INJECTIONS — 4

History of slimming syringes — 7

TYPES OF SLIMMING SYRINGES — 10

Latest approvals and market trends — 10
Types of weight loss syringes and their areas of application — 12
Dosage forms — 14
Manufacturer and distributor — 15
Novo Nordisk — 15
Eli Lilly and Company — 16
Orexigen Therapeutics (now part of Nalpropion Pharmaceuticals) — 16
Rhythm Pharmaceuticals — 17
AstraZeneca — 17
Sanofi — 17
Pfizer — 18
Boehringer Ingelheim and Eli Lilly — 18
Vivus Inc. — 18
Nalpropion Pharmaceuticals — 18
Eisai Co. — 19
Janssen Pharmaceuticals — 19
Merck & Co. — 19
Market leader — 20

THE SCIENCE BEHIND WEIGHT LOSS INJECTIONS — 22

How do weight loss injections work? — 23
Active ingredients and their mechanisms of action — 24
Comparison of the effectiveness of different weight loss injections — 26

SUCCESSES OF WEIGHT LOSS INJECTIONS — 28

CLINICAL STUDIES	**28**
STEP STUDY SERIES FOR SEMAGLUTIDE	**28**
SELECT STUDY FOR SEMAGLUTIDE	**30**
SCALE STUDY SERIES FOR LIRAGLUTIDE	**31**
SCALE OBESITY AND PREDIABETES	31
SCALE DIABETES	32
LIGHT STUDY FOR NALTREXONE-BUPROPION (CONTRAVE)	**34**
CONTRAVE	**35**

LONG-TERM EFFECTS AND SUSTAINABILITY OF WEIGHT LOSS — **38**

RISKS AND SIDE EFFECTS — **41**

COMMON SIDE EFFECTS	**41**
RARE SIDE EFFECTS	**42**
PANCREATITIS	42
GALLBLADDER DISEASES	44
KIDNEY PROBLEMS	45
THYROID CARCINOMA	47
DIABETIC RETINOPATHY	48
LONG-TERM HEALTH RISKS FROM WEIGHT LOSS INJECTIONS	**50**
RISKS FOR CERTAIN ORGAN SYSTEMS	50
LONG-TERM HORMONAL AND CELLULAR EFFECTS	51
RECOMMENDATIONS FOR LONG-TERM USE	51
RISKS FOR CERTAIN ORGAN SYSTEMS	**52**
LONG-TERM HORMONAL AND CELLULAR EFFECTS	**54**
CONTRAINDICATIONS	**57**
PRECAUTIONARY MEASURES	**60**
MIXTURE OF DIFFERENT MEDICATIONS	**61**

WHICH SLIMMING INJECTION FOR WHOM? — **63**

SELECTION BY PREPARATION	**63**
GLP-1 RECEPTOR AGONISTS (WEGOVY, SAXENDA, TRULICITY)	63
AMYLIN ANALOGUES (SYMLIN)	68
COMBINATION PREPARATIONS (CONTRAVE)	70

HEALTH STATUS AS A SELECTION CRITERION	72
INTERACTIONS WITH OTHER MEDICATIONS AS A CRITERION	73
SIDE EFFECTS AS A SELECTION CRITERION	74
LONG-TERM EFFECTS AS A SELECTION CRITERION	76
AVAILABILITY AS A SELECTION CRITERION	77
COST AS A SELECTION CRITERION	79
MARKET PRICES AND MANUFACTURERS	79
ADDITIONAL COSTS	80
INSURANCE COVER	80

OPTIMUM USE OF WEIGHT LOSS SYRINGES — 83

CORRECT APPLICATION AND DOSAGE	**83**
SELF-INJECTION TRAINING	83
SELECTION OF THE INJECTION SITE	84
DOSAGE INSTRUCTIONS	84
MONITORING AND CUSTOMISATION	85
COMBINATION WITH NUTRITION PLANS AND EXERCISE PROGRAMMES	**85**
NUTRITION PLANS	86
EXERCISE PROGRAMMES	87
REGULAR REVIEW AND ADJUSTMENT	87
MEDICAL MONITORING OF TREATMENT	88
TREATMENT DURATION	88
INTERRUPTION OF TREATMENT	90

SOURCES OF SUPPLY — 92

ETHICAL AND SOCIAL CONSIDERATIONS — 94

NEW DRUGS, CONCLUSION AND OUTLOOK — 97

Introduction to the topic of weight loss injections

We are getting fatter and fatter, and even beyond the associated health problems, we often don't like it. Our friends on YouTube and TikTok look much better. But what can we do? The tenth diet? Why should it work all at once?

The increasing problem of weight gain worldwide is known to be due to a variety of factors. Changing eating habits play a major role, as processed foods rich in sugar, fat and salt are becoming more readily available and often cheaper than healthy options. These foods lead to an increased calorie intake without being correspondingly nutritious.

At the same time, the lifestyle of many people has changed significantly. The modern world of work and leisure are increasingly characterised by sedentary activities, which greatly reduces physical activity. This lack of exercise is a decisive factor in the global increase in obesity.

Economic conditions also influence dietary behaviour. In many countries, healthy food is more expensive and harder to come by than fast food and other unhealthy options. Added to this is psychological stress, which often leads to increased eating behaviour, as many people use food to cope with stress. This emotional factor can be further exacerbated by the constant availability of food and the advertising of unhealthy foods.

The environment in which people live also plays a role. A lack of safe and accessible places for physical activity and an environment that encourages the consumption of unhealthy foods contribute to weight gain.

Many diets, on the other hand, regularly fail because they are often unrealistic and difficult to maintain. They often require drastic, unpleasant changes to the diet that are difficult to maintain in the long term. They can also lead to a feeling of deprivation, which increases the risk of food cravings. In addition, many diets focus on rapid weight loss rather than long-term dietary changes, which often leads to the so-called yo-yo effect, where the lost weight is quickly regained.

These framework conditions require a comprehensive and innovative approach to combating the epidemic. Weight loss injections are playing an increasingly important role in this.

These are, in short, medical injections used to aid weight loss. They are also known as weight loss injections or anti-obesity injections and are mainly prescribed to people who are overweight or obese, especially if there are associated health problems such as type 2 diabetes, high blood pressure or cardiovascular disease. Nowadays, however, weight loss injections are also increasingly being used to "simply lose weight", even if there are no strong medical indications.

The mode of action of these drugs is based on mimicking or enhancing hormones that are naturally present in the body and regulate food intake and energy metabolism. Many weight loss injections increase the feeling of satiety by delaying gastric emptying or acting directly on the centre of the brain responsible for the feeling of hunger. As a result, a person feels full faster, eats less and can lose weight more easily.

Weight loss injections have attracted a lot of attention in recent years, mainly because they enable clearly measurable weight loss, which has indeed been proven in clinical studies. Their effectiveness, combined with the ability to maintain the reduced weight in the long term, sets them apart from traditional dietary approaches. Awareness of these drugs has also increased through the use and recommendation of celebrities, which in turn has led to extensive media coverage - especially on social media channels. Here, uncontrolled growth is inevitable.

In addition, the increasing availability of these treatments, particularly through authorisations from health authorities and the possibility of prescribing via telemedicine or the internet, has contributed to more and more people having access to these medicines. This coincides with a growing public awareness of the health risks associated with obesity, such as diabetes and heart disease. Weight loss injections are therefore often seen as a hopeful option for those looking for effective weight management solutions. In short, if weight loss injections didn't already exist, they would have to be invented.

Ongoing research and development in this area also promises further improvements and innovations, which further increases scientific and public interest. All these factors together make weight loss injections a much-discussed topic that is seen by both medical experts and the general public as a potential breakthrough in the fight against the obesity epidemic.

History of slimming syringes

Slimming injections have not been around for long, they are relatively new developments that are only now becoming commonplace and therefore the subject of heated debate.

The story began in the late 20th century when scientists sought to discover and understand the hormonal and neurochemical pathways that regulate hunger and satiety. A pivotal moment in the history of this medical intervention was the discovery of glucagon-like peptide-1 (GLP-1), a hormone released by intestinal cells after eating that influences both insulin secretion and satiety.

Glucagon-like peptide-1 was discovered in the early 1980s. This discovery was part of a larger field of research investigating the gut and its role in regulating body physiology, particularly in relation to insulin secretion and glucose metabolism. GLP-1 belongs to a class of hormones known as incretins. These hormones are secreted by the gut after eating and play an important role in controlling the amount of insulin released by the pancreas in response to food intake.

The research that led to the identification of GLP-1 contributed significantly to the understanding of how the body regulates glucose levels and laid the foundation for the subsequent development of GLP-1 agonists as therapeutic agents against both type 2 diabetes and obesity.

The first medical trials with GLP-1 agonists initially focussed on diabetes treatment, but it soon became clear that these active ingredients also had the potential to help with weight loss.

Liraglutide was then developed by Novo Nordisk in 2005 and initially used to treat diabetes. Following further studies that confirmed its effectiveness in weight loss, it was approved in 2014 under the trade name Saxenda specifically for the treatment of obesity. This approval marked an important milestone in the history of weight loss injections, as it was one of the first drugs to be developed and approved specifically for this purpose.

Subsequent research and development led to further breakthroughs, including the introduction of semaglutide (Wegovy), which was approved by the US FDA in 2021 specifically for weight loss and showed even greater efficacy than previous drugs in clinical trials. These newer generations of weight loss injections offer improved dosing regimens and are even more targeted in their effects, making them a valuable tool in the fight against the obesity epidemic.

Thus, the initial discoveries in the field of endocrine physiology and the resulting medical innovations have laid the foundation for the development of today's weight loss injections. These advances reflect the scientific community's growing understanding of obesity as a multifactorial disease and the need for targeted, effective treatment.

Types of slimming syringes

The modern development and use of weight loss injections has been characterised by significant advances in biotechnology and pharmacology. These advances have led to the production of highly effective drugs that specifically target the body's hormonal systems to regulate hunger and improve insulin production. Current technology in the production of these drugs includes recombinant DNA technologies, advanced purification processes and improved formulations that allow for a longer half-life of the active ingredients and simplified applicability.

Latest approvals and market trends

GLP-1 receptor agonists, particularly semaglutide (marketed as **Wegovy**), have gained significant attention from the medical community and the public in recent years. This class of drugs works by mimicking the natural hormone GLP-1, which plays a central role in the body's glucose metabolism and appetite control mechanism. The effects of GLP-1 include enhancing insulin release in response to food intake, slowing gastric emptying and increasing satiety, which ultimately leads to reduced food intake.

Semaglutide is particularly in focus as it has shown weight loss benefits beyond what has been achieved with previous drugs in this class. Following its original approval as a diabetes treatment under the name **Ozempic**, semaglutide received approval under the name **Wegovy** specifically for the treatment of obesity in the US and Europe. The approval was based on extensive clinical trials that showed an average weight reduction of around 15% of body weight, a result rarely achieved in previous obesity therapies.

The popularity of semaglutide and other GLP-1 receptor agonists such as liraglutide (**Saxenda**) and dulaglutide (**Trulicity**) is also due to their relative safety and good tolerability. These drugs have a favourable side effect profile compared to many older weight loss drugs, making them a preferred choice for long-term use. These characteristics, together with good efficacy, have led to these drugs being seen as life-changing treatment options not only for people with obesity, but also for those suffering from weight-related health problems.

The increasing popularity of this class of drugs underlines the growing acceptance of pharmacological treatments for obesity, a disease that has traditionally been addressed through diet and exercise, but often requires additional therapeutic intervention to be treated effectively and sustainably.

These approvals underline the trend towards drugs developed specifically for long-term use in weight management programmes. The market for weight loss injections is growing as the prevalence of obesity increases worldwide and the need for effective treatment options increases.

Types of weight loss syringes and their areas of application

Developments in weight loss injections have led to a variety of treatment options that can be customised to the individual needs and medical conditions of patients. These developments reflect the advanced understanding of body mechanisms and hormone effects that researchers and physicians have gained over the years.

GLP-1 receptor agonists such as liraglutide and semaglutide are currently the leaders in this group and utilise the principle of the natural hormone GLP-1. This hormone is released after eating and works in a number of ways: It stimulates the release of insulin when blood glucose levels rise, delays gastric emptying and thus promotes a longer feeling of satiety, which in turn helps to reduce food intake. These effects make GLP-1 receptor agonists particularly effective in the treatment of obesity and have helped make them a popular choice for long-term weight management strategies.

Combination therapies such as the combination of **bupropion** and **naltrexone, known by** the trade name **Contrave**, offer a multi-mechanistic approach. **Bupropion** is an antidepressant that is also used for smoking cessation and is known to have appetite suppressant effects, while **naltrexone** was originally used to treat opioid and alcohol dependence. This combination aims to influence neurochemical pathways in the brain that control cravings and reward centres, while increasing feelings of satiety. This makes **Contrave** an effective tool for people who have difficulty controlling their eating habits.

Research into other hormone therapies that focus on modulating the effects of cortisol offers an innovative approach in the fight against obesity, particularly with regard to stress-induced weight gain. **Cortisol**, often referred to as the "stress hormone", plays a central role in the body's stress response system. Under chronic stress, increased cortisol production can lead to various metabolic changes, including increased appetite, weight gain and unfavourable fat distribution, typically around the abdominal area.

Therapies that target the regulation of **cortisol** could potentially reduce the negative effects of stress on body weight. These approaches would not only directly influence cortisol levels, but also act on the complex interactions between stress, hunger and fat metabolism. This could be an effective way to reduce stress-induced food cravings and overeating and thus control weight gain.

The development of such therapies is particularly relevant at a time when many people are exposed to increased psychological and social stress, which often leads to unhealthy eating habits and ultimately obesity. By addressing the biochemical pathways that are influenced by **cortisol,** one could provide a multidimensional treatment strategy that takes into account not only physiological but also psychological aspects of obesity.

However, research in this area is still relatively new and the challenges in developing such therapies include accurately determining dosage, avoiding side effects and customising treatment to achieve optimal results. Nevertheless, the potential of these therapeutic approaches to improve the quality of life of those affected and reduce the healthcare costs associated with obesity and stress-related diseases makes them a promising field of research in medical science.

Dosage forms

Slimming injections usually come in the form of subcutaneous injections that patients can administer themselves. This dosage form has proven to be effective because it allows for a controlled release of the active ingredient and ensures direct absorption into the bloodstream. Here are some details on the common dosage forms and their application:

- Pre-filled pen or injector: Many weight loss syringes, such as those containing GLP-1 receptor agonists (e.g. liraglutide, semaglutide), are offered in the form of a pre-filled pen or injector. These pens are easy to use and allow patients to inject themselves with minimal training. The pens are usually equipped with a fine needle, which makes the injection less painful.
- Dosage and frequency of use: Most slimming injections are administered once a day or once a week. The exact dosage and frequency of

administration depends on the specific medication and the individual needs of the patient. For example, liraglutide is injected daily, while semaglutide and tirzepatide are usually administered once a week.
- Instructions for self-injection: When first prescribed, patients usually receive detailed instructions from a healthcare provider on how to carry out the injection correctly. This includes instructions on how to store the medication, how to prepare the injection and how to dispose of the needles.

By using these forms of injections, active ingredients can be efficiently delivered into the body, leading to significant weight loss in many cases. The self-administration of these injections also offers a convenient option for patients who may have difficulty attending regular medical appointments.

Manufacturer and distributor

Various pharmaceutical companies develop and market slimming injections based on specific mechanisms of action. Here is an overview of some of the best-known manufacturers and the products they offer:

Novo Nordisk

- **Saxenda (liraglutide)**: Originally developed for the treatment of type 2 diabetes (under the name

Victoza), Saxenda is specifically approved for weight loss in adults with a BMI of 30 or more or 27 or more with at least one weight-related comorbidity.
- **Wegovy (semaglutide)**: A higher dose of the active ingredient semaglutide, also known as **Ozempic,** for the treatment of type 2 diabetes. Wegovy is specifically approved for chronic weight management therapy.
- **Ozempic (semaglutide)**: Although primarily approved for the treatment of type 2 diabetes, Ozempic has also shown that it can lead to significant measurable weight loss. In many cases, Ozempic was used off-label for weight loss before it was approved specifically for this purpose under the name Wegovy.

Eli Lilly and Company

- **Trulicity (dulaglutide)**: Although primarily approved as a diabetes treatment, Trulicity is also effective for weight loss and is used for this purpose in some cases.

Orexigen Therapeutics (now part of Nalpropion Pharmaceuticals)

- **Contrave (bupropion and naltrexone)**: This medication combines two active ingredients with different mechanisms aimed at reducing appetite and increasing the feeling of fullness. It is specifically authorised for weight management.

Rhythm Pharmaceuticals

- **Imcivree (setmelanotide)**: This is a specific treatment approach for patients with rare genetic disorders of obesity. Imcivree is approved for the treatment of adults and children aged 6 years and older with certain genetic disorders that lead to obesity.

AstraZeneca

- **Bydureon (exenatide)**: This is a form of the GLP-1 receptor agonist exenatide, which is used for the treatment of type 2 diabetes but can also have positive effects on weight loss. Bydureon is usually injected once a week.

Sanofi

- **Soliqua/Suliqua (insulin glargine and lixisenatide)**: This combination product, which includes both a long-acting insulin and a GLP-1 receptor agonist, is used to treat type 2 diabetes but can also help with weight loss.

Pfizer

- **Rybelsus (semaglutide oral)**: This is an oral formulation of semaglutide that is approved for the treatment of type 2 diabetes. Like **Ozempic**, Rybelsus can also support weight loss, although it is not specifically marketed for this indication.

Boehringer Ingelheim and Eli Lilly

- **Jardiance (empagliflozin)**: Originally developed to treat type 2 diabetes, this SGLT2 inhibitor drug has shown that it can also contribute to weight loss, especially in patients with diabetes.

Vivus Inc.

- **Qsymia (phentermine and topiramate)**: Qsymia combines phentermine, an appetite suppressant, with topiramate, a drug originally developed to treat epilepsy that also promotes feelings of fullness. This drug is specifically approved for weight loss and is often used in patients who are not only overweight but also have co-morbidities such as hypertension or type 2 diabetes.

Nalpropion Pharmaceuticals

- **Contrave** (bupropion and naltrexone): As mentioned above, Contrave combines two active ingredients for weight loss. Originally developed by Orexigen Therapeutics, it is now marketed by Nalpropion Pharmaceuticals.

Eisai Co.

- **Belviq (lorcaserin):** This drug, which affects the activity of serotonin receptors in the brain to increase feelings of satiety, was approved in the US for weight loss but was withdrawn from the market due to concerns about possible cancer risks.

Janssen Pharmaceuticals

- **Invokana (canagliflozin):** An SGLT2 inhibitor originally developed for the treatment of type 2 diabetes. Like other SGLT2 inhibitors, Invokana can also contribute to weight loss by causing the body to excrete excess sugar via the urine.

Merck & Co.

- **Steglatro (ertugliflozin):** Also an SGLT2 inhibitor that is approved for the treatment of type 2 diabetes and offers potential weight loss benefits.

These and other companies and their products demonstrate the range of approaches and mechanisms that are now available for the treatment of overweight and obesity.

Market leader

Novo Nordisk and Eli Lilly are currently the leading companies in the market for weight loss injections, particularly in the category of GLP-1 receptor agonists specifically designed for weight loss. Novo Nordisk, a Danish pharmaceutical company, has a significant influence in the field of weight management therapies with products such as **Saxenda** and **Wegovy**.

Eli Lilly, based in the US, competes closely with Novo Nordisk and has shown strong market presence with **Trulicity,** which also enables significant weight loss. In addition, Eli Lilly is developing **Tirzepatide, which is considered a** breakthrough in the industry due to its potentially high weight loss efficacy and could soon play a major role in the market. **Tirzepatide is** an innovative drug that shows particular promise for the treatment of type 2 diabetes and obesity. As a dual GIP and GLP-1 receptor agonist, tirzepatide simulates the effects of two incretin hormones, allowing it to both regulate blood glucose levels and increase satiety. This leads to improved control of blood glucose levels and a significant reduction in weight.

The particular combination of effects that **tirzepatide** offers, namely supporting insulin secretion based on blood glucose levels and simultaneously reducing food intake by increasing satiety, makes the drug particularly valuable in the future. These properties are crucial as many people with type 2 diabetes also struggle with overweight or obesity, and treatment that effectively addresses both conditions can significantly improve health and reduce the risk of diabetes-related complications.

The results from the clinical trials have particularly impressed the medical community, as **tirzepatide** not only showed better efficacy in blood glucose control than existing GLP-1 receptor agonists, but also led to remarkable weight loss. This potential places **tirzepatide at** the centre of hopes for a new generation of diabetes and weight management therapies that could both improve quality of life and provide more comprehensive and effective treatment options for patients. The combination of therapeutic effects in a single drug offers a significant advance and symbolises the progress in pharmaceutical research that could revolutionise the management of metabolic disease.

Novo Nordisk and Eli Lilly have already achieved a dominant position by developing effective and safe medicines for obesity and diabetes and continue to invest significantly in research and development to open up new treatment options. Their leadership is also strengthened by extensive clinical trials and a strong global presence, helping to shape the market for weight management therapies.

The science behind weight loss injections

Weight loss injections utilise complex physiological processes to both reduce appetite and influence insulin production, making them an effective method for weight management and the treatment of metabolic diseases. In particular, the group of GLP-1 receptor agonists, which are frequently used in these medications, play a central role.

These drugs mimic the effect of naturally occurring hormones such as glucagon-like peptide-1 (GLP-1). GLP-1 is produced in the small intestine after food intake and is crucial for the regulation of blood glucose levels and appetite. By binding to GLP-1 receptors, these drugs stimulate insulin release from the pancreas in a glucose-dependent manner, i.e. insulin secretion is increased when blood glucose levels rise, preventing overproduction of insulin and associated hypoglycaemia. At the same time, gastric emptying is delayed, which keeps the patient fuller for longer and thus reduces calorie consumption throughout the day.

In addition, these hormones have a direct effect on the brain, where they influence appetite regulation. They activate certain areas in the brain that are responsible for the feeling of satiety, which reduces the feeling of hunger and leads to a lower calorie intake. This dual approach - improving the insulin response and controlling the feeling of hunger - makes GLP-1 receptor agonists particularly effective in the treatment of obesity and type 2 diabetes.

The ability of these drugs to mimic and enhance the body's natural mechanisms provides an effective and relatively safe way to treat weight problems that prove difficult to treat through conventional methods such as diet and exercise alone. These properties explain why they are increasingly recognised as an important part of therapeutic strategies for obesity and related metabolic disorders.

How do slimming syringes work?

GLP-1 receptor agonists, a major group of weight loss injections, utilise a very effective principle by mimicking the body's natural processes that become active after food intake. By simulating the GLP-1 hormone, they achieve a multiple effect that affects both metabolism and appetite, making them an effective tool in the management of obesity and type 2 diabetes.

The hormone GLP-1, which is naturally produced in the lower small intestine after food intake, plays a central role in regulating blood sugar levels. It stimulates the pancreas to release more insulin when blood sugar levels rise, which helps to effectively lower blood sugar. This insulinotropic effect only occurs in the presence of elevated glucose levels, which reduces the risk of unwanted hypoglycaemia that can occur with other diabetes treatments.

In addition to influencing insulin secretion, GLP-1 also slows gastric emptying, resulting in prolonged satiety after meals, thus reducing appetite and food intake. This delay in gastric emptying helps to mitigate blood glucose spikes after meals, contributing to more stable glycaemic control overall.

In addition, GLP-1 directly influences the central nervous system by acting on certain areas of the brain that are responsible for the regulation of hunger and satiety. By activating these areas of the brain, the feeling of hunger and the associated behaviours that lead to food intake are reduced.

This multi-faceted mode of action makes GLP-1 receptor agonists particularly attractive for the treatment of patients in whom both weight management and glycaemic control play a role. By addressing multiple fronts simultaneously, these drugs offer a comprehensive strategy for the treatment of obesity and type 2 diabetes.

Active ingredients and their mechanisms of action

GLP-1 receptor agonists such as liraglutide and semaglutide play the central role already described in the modern treatment of diabetes and obesity by binding specifically to GLP-1 receptors in the body.

This binding leads to increased insulin secretion, which is only activated when blood glucose levels are elevated, significantly reducing the risk of hypoglycaemia, a common problem with other diabetes medications. In addition, they slow down gastric emptying, which prolongs the feeling of satiety and thus reduces food intake. These properties make them an effective option for weight management and diabetes control.

In contrast, combination preparations such as bupropion and naltrexone, known under the trade name Contrave, combine different mechanisms of action that influence eating behaviour. Bupropion, an antidepressant, inhibits appetite by modulating the neurotransmitters dopamine and noradrenaline. Naltrexone interferes with the brain's reward system to reduce the urge to eat. This combination works synergistically to reduce food cravings and modify eating habits.

In practice, GLP-1 receptor agonists often show a greater effect on weight loss compared to combination drugs. Drugs such as semaglutide can achieve an average weight reduction of around 15% of body weight in clinical trials, making them particularly effective for people who need significant weight loss. Contrave and similar combination therapies can also be effective, especially in patients whose eating behaviour is strongly influenced by psychological factors such as stress and reward behaviour.

The selection of the appropriate medication depends heavily on the individual's health conditions, the presence of comorbidities such as type 2 diabetes and the patient's specific needs and goals. Both classes of medication offer valuable options for the management of weight and diabetes, but in different contexts and with different efficacy profiles. More on this in detail later.

Comparison of the effectiveness of different weight loss injections

The effectiveness of slimming injections varies depending on the composition of the active ingredient and the individual patient's reaction.

GLP-1 receptor agonists, such as semaglutide and liraglutide, have been shown to be particularly effective in clinical trials, especially semaglutide, which is marketed in higher doses for specific weight loss under the name Wegovy. Semaglutide often achieves an average weight loss of around 15% of body weight in these studies, while liraglutide and similar drugs usually result in a weight loss of 5-10%.

In comparison, combination drugs such as Contrave, which combines bupropion and naltrexone, offer a different therapeutic option. These medications are particularly suitable for patients whose eating behaviour is strongly influenced by psychological factors such as stress eating. Although they can be effective, practice shows that their effectiveness in terms of weight reduction is often lower than that of GLP-1 receptor agonists. However, Contrave and similar combination therapies are useful for patients who benefit from treatment that addresses both physical and emotional food cravings.

These different efficacy profiles mean that choosing the right weight loss injection requires careful consideration, taking into account not only the patient's individual health goals and medical conditions, but also their personal response to treatment. For example, patients who suffer from type 2 diabetes as well as being overweight may particularly benefit from GLP-1 receptor agonists, while those with a strong psychological component to their eating behaviour may achieve better results with a combination drug.

Overall, weight loss injections offer an effective method of weight loss that works through a combination of appetite control and improved metabolic function. However, the choice of specific medication should always be made in conjunction with a healthcare professional to ensure the best and safest option for the individual patient.

Success of weight loss injections

Clinical studies

The efficacy and safety of weight loss injections, particularly GLP-1 receptor agonists, have been well documented in numerous clinical studies. These studies have shown that these drugs are not only effective in weight loss, but can also reduce the risk of obesity-related diseases.

STEP study series for semaglutide

- The STEP 1 study focussed on weight loss in adults with obesity or overweight and investigated the efficacy of semaglutide compared to a placebo, supplemented with lifestyle interventions. In this study, participants were given either semaglutide or a placebo, and both groups were encouraged to improve their diet and exercise habits at the same time. The results of the study were remarkable: those who received semaglutide experienced an average weight loss of about 14.9% of their body weight. This represents a success and highlights the potential effectiveness of semaglutide as a weight loss aid, especially when combined with lifestyle changes.
- The STEP 2 study aimed to investigate the effects of semaglutide on adults with type 2 diabetes. In

this study, the efficacy of semaglutide was evaluated not only in terms of weight loss, but also in terms of its ability to improve glycaemic control. Participants receiving semaglutide experienced significant improvements in both glycaemic control and body weight. These results confirm the dual efficacy of semaglutide, which not only serves as a weight loss agent, but can also play an important role in diabetes management by helping to effectively manage blood glucose levels.

- The STEP 3 study was specifically designed to investigate the sustainability of weight loss achieved with semaglutide. In this phase of the study, all participants initially received semaglutide for 20 weeks to observe the immediate effects of the drug on body weight. This initial phase was followed by a longer observation period of 48 weeks, during which half of the participants continued to receive semaglutide, while the other half were switched to a placebo. This study design allowed the researchers to observe not only the short-term effects of semaglutide on weight loss, but also to evaluate how well weight loss was maintained over a longer period of time when treatment was continued compared to when it was discontinued. The results showed that participants who continued to receive semaglutide were able to effectively maintain their reduced weight, while those who switched to placebo tended to regain weight. These findings are particularly valuable as they emphasise the importance of continued treatment with semaglutide for the long-term maintenance of weight loss. They confirm that although initial weight loss is an important step, continued use of semaglutide may be crucial to maintain the health benefits achieved and counteract any potential weight regain.

SELECT study for semaglutide

The SELECT study is a comprehensive clinical trial investigating the long-term cardiovascular and metabolic effects of semaglutide in people with obesity without diabetes. This study is particularly important as it aims to determine whether semaglutide can reduce the risk of serious cardiovascular events in a population that is overweight but not affected by type 2 diabetes. Cardiovascular disease is closely linked to obesity and is a major cause of morbidity and mortality globally. Therefore, a positive result from this study could have important implications for the treatment of obesity.

The SELECT study is designed as a double-blind, placebo-controlled, randomised trial to minimise errors and ensure the integrity of the data. Participants from different countries are observed over an extended period of time, during which semaglutide or a placebo is administered. This methodological approach will allow the researchers to collect reliable data on how semaglutide affects the risk of cardiovascular events.

The importance of the results of this study cannot be overestimated. If the final data show that semaglutide can reduce cardiovascular risk in obese patients without diabetes, this could have a significant impact on obesity treatment strategies. Such a result would lead to a broader use of GLP-1 receptor agonists in this patient group and fundamentally change and expand the therapeutic approaches for obesity.

In addition, a better understanding of the cardiovascular effects of semaglutide would help to improve the safety profile of this class of drugs. By gaining information on potential risks and benefits, the study could help optimise treatment to ensure not only efficacy but also patient safety and well-being. Such research is crucial to making informed clinical decisions and improving the overall health and quality of life of people with obesity.

SCALE study series for liraglutide

SCALE Obesity and Prediabetes

The SCALE Obesity and Prediabetes study investigated the effectiveness of liraglutide in the context of weight loss in people with obesity and prediabetes. The results of this study were very informative regarding the potential benefits of liraglutide for this specific patient group.

In the study, participants received either liraglutide or a placebo. The data showed that a significant number of people who received liraglutide experienced substantial weight loss. Specifically, 63% of participants treated with liraglutide lost at least 5% of their body weight. In comparison, only 27% of participants in the placebo group achieved this weight loss.

This significant difference in results emphasises the efficacy of liraglutide as a weight loss aid in people with obesity and prediabetes. It should be noted that a weight loss of at least 5% in people with obesity and prediabetes may not only provide aesthetic or physical benefits, but may also sustainably reduce the risk of developing type 2 diabetes and other metabolic diseases.

The SCALE study thus provides important findings that can be used in medical practice to improve treatment strategies for patients with prediabetes and obesity. Such results are important for the development of targeted interventions that not only reduce weight, but also improve overall health and well-being.

SCALE Diabetes

The SCALE Diabetes study focused on the effects of liraglutide on people with type 2 diabetes, particularly in terms of weight reduction and improved glycaemic control. Liraglutide is a GLP-1 receptor agonist that was originally developed for the treatment of type 2 diabetes and was also investigated in this study for its ability to reduce weight.

The results of the SCALE Diabetes study showed that treatment with liraglutide not only led to measurable weight loss, but also improved blood glucose control in the participants. This is particularly relevant as both obesity and poor glycaemic control are among the main factors that increase the risk of complications of diabetes, such as cardiovascular disease, kidney damage and retinopathy.

The improved glycaemic control provided by liraglutide is likely due to several mechanisms, including the stimulation of insulin secretion in response to elevated blood glucose levels and the delay in gastric emptying, resulting in a slower and steadier influx of glucose into the blood. These effects help to reduce post-meal blood glucose spikes, which is a critical aspect in the treatment of type 2 diabetes.

Weight loss in people with type 2 diabetes with liraglutide can offer additional benefits, as weight loss often leads to improved insulin sensitivity. This means that the body's cells respond better to insulin and can absorb glucose from the bloodstream more efficiently, further helping to lower blood glucose levels.

In summary, the SCALE Diabetes study provides valuable insights into how liraglutide can contribute not only to glycaemic control but also to weight management in people with type 2 diabetes as part of a comprehensive treatment plan.

LIGHT study for naltrexone-bupropion (Contrave)

The LIGHT study was an important clinical investigation aimed at evaluating the effects of the drug naltrexone-bupropion on cardiovascular risk in overweight and obese patients. Naltrexone-bupropion is a combination therapy often prescribed for weight loss as it can reduce food cravings and increase satiety. Investigating the cardiovascular risk profile of this drug was crucial, as overweight and obesity are themselves risk factors for cardiovascular disease.

Although the LIGHT trial was terminated prematurely, it still provided important insights into the safety of naltrexone-bupropion. Such premature terminations are not uncommon in the world of clinical research and still offer important learning opportunities.

The safety data collected during the study is of great importance as it will help physicians and patients make informed decisions about the use of naltrexone bupropion for weight loss, especially in patients with existing cardiovascular conditions or at high risk for such conditions. These data can shed light on whether the drug potentially increases the risk of heart attacks, strokes or other serious cardiovascular events.

In conclusion, the results of the LIGHT study have provided valuable information on the safety profile of naltrexone-bupropion, despite its early discontinuation. This information is crucial for the further development of treatment guidelines and may help to make the management of patients seeking drug support for weight loss safer.

Contrave

Contrave was also evaluated in clinical studies, which showed that it can effectively reduce body weight.

Contrave was developed specifically for weight loss and has shown positive results in clinical trials. The active ingredient bupropion is known for its antidepressant properties and ability to suppress tobacco cravings, while naltrexone is mainly used in the treatment of opioid and alcohol addictions. The combination of these two active ingredients aims to influence both the physiological and psychological aspects of food intake.

In one of the clinical studies on Contrave, participants who took the drug for a year lost an average of around 5% of their body weight. This compares to only about 1% weight loss in participants taking a placebo. This significant difference emphasises the effectiveness of Contrave in supporting weight loss.

A key benefit of Contrave is its ability to reduce food cravings and improve control over eating behaviour. This is particularly valuable for people who have a strong psychological attachment to food, such as those who eat for emotional reasons or have difficulty regulating their satiety appropriately. Contrave's mode of action can help break the cycles of cravings and overeating, which promotes sustainable weight loss.

In addition, the psychological effects of bupropion, such as improving mood and reducing depression, can help patients feel more motivated and less stressed during the weight loss process. This can be a crucial factor in long-term weight loss success and maintaining a healthy lifestyle.

Thus, Contrave offers an effective solution for weight management by acting on both physiological and psychological factors that influence eating behaviour. This dual mode of action makes it a valuable tool for individuals who have difficulty controlling their weight through diet and exercise alone.

These studies are just a small sample of a large body of research dedicated to evaluating the safety, efficacy and long-term effects of these drugs. They are helping to define and refine the therapeutic applications of weight loss injections to ensure that they are both effective and safe for the patients who need them.

They demonstrate not only the effectiveness of these drugs in weight loss, but also their potential to provide further health benefits by reducing risk factors for chronic diseases such as type 2 diabetes and cardiovascular disease. These results have contributed significantly to the recognition of weight loss injections as safe and effective treatment options for obesity and overweight.

Long-term effects and sustainability of weight reduction

The use of weight loss injections has established itself as an effective method in recent years, especially for people who have difficulty losing weight through diet and exercise alone.

The long-term effects of weight loss injections based on the action of GLP-1 receptor agonists are another important aspect of their popularity and effectiveness. The continuous support provided by these drugs can help to change eating behaviour in the long term. Patients often learn to eat smaller portions and feel fuller more quickly, which helps to improve and stabilise weight management. This mechanism also helps to avoid the yo-yo effect that often occurs after the end of traditional diets, as the original eating behaviour is often quickly resumed.

The sustained effectiveness of these treatments is further supported by studies that show that patients who use this therapy in the long term can experience consistent weight loss or successful weight stabilisation. However, it is important that the use of such injections is seen as part of a holistic approach that also includes lifestyle changes and psychological support where appropriate.

It is therefore not only the direct effect on eating behaviour and metabolism that promotes the sustainability of these treatments, but also the guidance and motivation for a healthier lifestyle that can be maintained in the long term.

The duration of use of weight loss injections can vary greatly and is significantly influenced by the patient's individual response to treatment and the occurrence of side effects. Drugs such as GLP-1 receptor agonists are generally designed for long-term treatment, and many clinical studies support their use over several years as long as patients benefit and the treatment is well tolerated.

The question of the duration of use is also not always easy to answer because obesity is seen as a chronic disease that requires a continuous and long-term management strategy. Current medical guidelines often recommend that such drug therapies should be used as part of a comprehensive treatment plan that is continued even after the target weight has been reached in order to maintain the successes achieved and prevent regaining weight.

The integration of lifestyle changes is an important aspect of these treatments. Medication support can help to facilitate the necessary adjustments in diet and exercise behaviour by reducing hunger and promoting satiety. In the long term, however, the aim is for patients to internalise these behavioural changes and maintain them even without medication support.

When the use of weight loss injections is discontinued, it is important that the learned behaviours of healthy eating and regular physical activity are maintained. Without these continued efforts, there is a real risk of relapsing into old patterns and thus regaining weight. Therefore, the decision to stop treatment should always be made carefully and ideally in consultation with a healthcare professional to ensure a planned transition and ongoing support.

The long-term use of slimming injections is therefore generally sensible, but naturally requires continuous medical monitoring. This is necessary in order to monitor possible side effects or long-term complications. The most common side effects include nausea, vomiting, diarrhoea and possible irritation at the injection site. More serious but rare risks can include pancreatitis, gallbladder disease and even rare forms of thyroid cancer.

For effective and sustainable weight loss, these injections should ultimately be used as an important part of a comprehensive treatment plan. This plan should also include dietary changes, regular physical activity and psychological support. The combination of these measures will not only reduce weight, but also minimise the risk of weight gain in the future.

Risks and side effects

Weight loss injections are an increasingly popular and often very useful method of supporting weight loss. However, the use of these drugs also harbours potential side effects and risks that can be relevant in both the short and long term.

Common side effects

Weight loss injections, especially those based on GLP-1 receptor agonists, often lead to gastrointestinal complaints.

It can take a while for the body to adapt to the medication, and during this time symptoms such as nausea, vomiting, diarrhoea and constipation may occur. These effects often diminish after a familiarisation period as the body develops a certain tolerance to the drug. This is an important aspect for patients to keep in mind, as good symptom control and lifestyle adjustments can help to better manage the initial phase of treatment.

In addition to the digestive problems, headaches, dizziness and an increased heart rate can occur as side effects. These symptoms are also part of the body's adaptation response to the medication. Headaches and dizziness may be caused by changes in blood circulation and hydration induced by the medication. The increased heart rate may be caused by the stimulating effect of the drug on the cardiovascular system.

It is very important that patients who experience these side effects receive close medical care. Regular monitoring by healthcare providers helps to keep an eye on the side effects and to react in good time if adjustments to the therapy are necessary. This may include adjusting the dose or changing the medication, especially if the side effects persist or are particularly troublesome.

Close co-operation with the attending physician is therefore essential to ensure safe and effective treatment. If necessary, the doctor can make therapeutic adjustments to improve the tolerability of the medication and increase the patient's quality of life during treatment.

Rare side effects

The rare side effects of drugs containing GLP-1 receptor agonists can be serious and cause long-term health problems.

Pancreatitis

The link between the use of GLP-1 receptor agonists and the occurrence of pancreatitis is a critical issue in the consideration of these weight loss drugs.

Pancreatitis, an inflammation of the pancreas, is a potentially life-threatening condition that can be acute or chronic. Symptoms of acute pancreatitis include severe abdominal pain, nausea, vomiting, fever and a rapid pulse. Chronic pancreatitis can lead to persistent abdominal pain, indigestion and even diabetes as the pancreas becomes damaged over time.

The exact mechanisms by which GLP-1 receptor agonists could cause pancreatitis are not yet fully understood. Some theories suggest that these drugs may affect the secretion of digestive enzymes, leading to premature activation of these enzymes and attacking the pancreas. It could also play a role that the drugs impair blood flow to the pancreas, which could lead to inflammation.

For patients with a history of pancreatic disease or those who have risk factors for pancreatitis (such as certain dietary habits or alcohol consumption), the use of GLP-1 receptor agonists should be considered with particular caution. These patients should be closely monitored and immediate medical action should be taken at the first sign of symptoms suggestive of possible pancreatitis.

The decision to use these medications should always be based on an individual risk-benefit assessment, taking into account the patient's health history, possible weight loss alternatives and the severity of obesity. Careful monitoring during therapy is essential to ensure the patient's well-being and to recognise and treat serious complications such as pancreatitis at an early stage.

Gallbladder diseases

Gallbladder disease is another possible side effect of using weight loss injections, especially in conjunction with rapid weight loss processes. Gallstones and cholecystitis (an inflammation of the gallbladder) are two common conditions that can occur in this context.

Gallstones form when solid particles accumulate and harden in the bile. These stones can vary in size and composition, with cholesterol stones being the most common. The gallbladder is used to store bile, which is produced by the liver and is needed to digest fat. If you lose a lot of weight, the composition of the bile can change, which favours the formation of gallstones. If weight loss is very rapid, this can increase the risk because the gallbladder is emptied less frequently and the bile remains in the gallbladder for longer, increasing the likelihood of stone formation.

Cholecystitis occurs when gallstones block the outflow of bile, leading to inflammation. This blockage can cause severe pain in the upper right abdomen, fever and vomiting. Untreated cholecystitis can lead to more serious complications, including rupture of the gallbladder.

Treatment of gallbladder disease often involves the management of pain medications and, in some cases, removal of the gallbladder through a surgical procedure known as cholecystectomy. Prevention of gallstones and cholecystitis in patients on weight loss therapy with GLP-1 receptor agonists may require a less aggressive weight loss strategy to avoid abrupt changes in the gallbladder.

For patients using weight loss injections who are at risk for gallbladder disease, it may be advisable to moderate the weight loss process and choose a diet that includes regular meals to regularly empty the gallbladder. Close medical monitoring is also important in order to be able to react early to signs of gallbladder disease.

Kidney problems

Kidney problems are another issue with the use of GLP-1 receptor agonists, especially for people who already suffer from impaired kidney function. These drugs can affect kidney function and exacerbate existing kidney problems.

The kidneys play a central role in the filtration and elimination of waste products from the blood and in the regulation of fluid and electrolyte balance. Deterioration of kidney function can lead to a build-up of toxins in the body, which can cause a variety of health problems.

The possible mechanisms by which GLP-1 receptor agonists can cause or exacerbate kidney problems include

- Dehydration: Side effects such as nausea and vomiting can lead to fluid loss, which puts a strain on the kidneys.

- Altered blood circulation: The medication can affect the blood circulation in the kidneys, which can impair kidney function.
- Direct toxicity: There is evidence that some GLP-1 receptor agonists may have direct toxic effects on kidney cells.

For patients who already suffer from renal dysfunction, it is important to carefully monitor kidney function while being treated with GLP-1 receptor agonists. This includes regular blood tests to check kidney function, particularly blood creatinine and urea levels, and urinalyses to assess protein excretion and other kidney functions.

A deterioration in kidney function during treatment may require that the dose of the medication be adjusted or the treatment discontinued altogether. In addition, measures should be taken to ensure adequate hydration and minimise risk factors that can lead to kidney strain.

In cases where deterioration in kidney function is detected, a full assessment should be carried out by a nephrologist or appropriate specialist to discuss appropriate treatment options and minimise the risk of further damage. This emphasises the importance of holistic care and careful monitoring of patients using these potentially life-changing medications.

Thyroid carcinoma

The increased risk of thyroid cancer, particularly medullary thyroid carcinoma, with the use of GLP-1 receptor agonists is another side effect that is as serious as it is rare and requires special attention. These concerns stem from preclinical studies in which an increased rate of thyroid tumours was observed in rodents treated with GLP-1 receptor agonists. Although such findings are not always directly translatable to humans, this has led to increased vigilance and caution when prescribing these drugs.

Medullary thyroid carcinoma is a rare form of thyroid cancer that arises from the parafollicular cells (C-cells) of the thyroid gland. This type of cancer can be aggressive and difficult to treat once it has spread. The link between GLP-1 receptor agonists and the risk of medullary thyroid cancer is seen as a potential direct stimulation of cell growth by the drug.

For patients with a family history of medullary thyroid carcinoma or who suffer from multiple endocrine neoplasia type 2 (MEN 2), the use of GLP-1 receptor agonists is generally not recommended. MEN 2 is a genetic disorder associated with a high risk of medullary thyroid carcinoma and other endocrine disorders.

Patients being treated with GLP-1 receptor agonists should be made aware of possible symptoms of thyroid problems, such as swelling or lumps in the throat, hoarseness, difficulty swallowing or breathing problems. Regular thyroid examinations can be part of the monitoring plan, especially for patients at increased risk.

It can therefore be said that the potential risk of thyroid cancer is a serious consideration when using GLP-1 receptor agonists and requires careful consideration of the risk-benefit ratio by the treating physician, especially in high-risk groups.

Diabetic retinopathy

Diabetic retinopathy is another serious complication of diabetes that is caused by damage to the blood vessels of the retina and can lead to vision loss. While GLP-1 receptor agonists are primarily used for the treatment of type 2 diabetes and weight loss and have many positive effects on blood glucose levels and overall metabolic profile, there are reports suggesting an association between the use of these drugs and the development or worsening of diabetic retinopathy.

The exact mechanisms by which GLP-1 receptor agonists may contribute to retinopathy are not fully understood. One theory suggests that rapid changes in blood glucose levels, which can be caused by the strong blood glucose-lowering effect of GLP-1 receptor agonists, could lead to destabilisation of the retinal blood vessels. Another possibility could be that the drugs have indirect effects on the vascular system, leading to a deterioration in retinal health.

Because of these potential risks, it is important that patients using GLP-1 receptor agonists who already have type 2 diabetes are regularly examined by an ophthalmologist. This usually includes annual fundus examinations. This involves examining the back of the eye for signs of damage to the blood vessels. An optical coherence tomography (OCT), an imaging examination that provides detailed images of the structures of the eye and can recognise early signs of damage, may also be performed.

For patients with existing eye disease or those who have risk factors for developing diabetic retinopathy, these examinations may be required more frequently. It is also advisable that all patients using GLP-1 receptor agonists are informed of the symptoms of diabetic retinopathy, such as blurred vision, difficulty seeing colours, darkening or blank areas in the field of vision and sudden appearance of spots or "floating" dots that may indicate bleeding in the eye.

Regular monitoring and early detection can minimise the risks of serious visual impairment and initiate appropriate treatment if necessary.

Given these rare but potentially serious side effects, it is important that both doctors and patients are well informed and carry out regular health checks to ensure that treatment remains safe. If there are any signs of these serious side effects, medical help should be sought immediately and treatment should be adjusted accordingly.

Long-term health risks from weight loss injections

Long-term use of weight loss injections, particularly those containing GLP-1 receptor agonists, may pose potential health risks that should be considered when making treatment decisions. These drugs work by stimulating the GLP-1 receptor, resulting in improved insulin secretion, reduced glucagon release and delayed gastric emptying. These mechanisms not only support weight loss, but also have effects on various organ systems that lead to concerns with long-term use.

Risks for certain organ systems

- Renal function: As already mentioned, GLP-1 receptor agonists can exert additional stress on the kidneys in people with pre-existing renal impairment. The possible mechanisms for this include dehydration through nausea or vomiting and direct effects on kidney function. Long-term use could increase the risk of kidney damage, necessitating regular monitoring of kidney function.
- Pancreatitis: The risk of chronic or recurrent pancreatitis is also a serious consideration, especially for patients with a history of this condition. Stimulation of the GLP-1 receptor could potentially

lead to a change in the secretion of digestive enzymes, which may increase the risk of inflammation.

Long-term hormonal and cellular effects

- Hormonal balance: Chronic use of GLP-1 receptor agonists affects hormonal balance, particularly the hormones associated with glucose metabolism. This could have long-term effects on metabolism, the full consequences of which are not yet known.
- Cell growth regulation: Some studies suggest that long-term stimulation of the GLP-1 receptor may affect the growth of certain cell types, potentially increasing the risk of certain cancers, such as medullary thyroid carcinoma. These concerns are based primarily on animal studies and require further research to understand their relevance in humans.

Recommendations for long-term use

Because of these potential risks, it is generally recommended that the use of GLP-1 receptor agonists be carefully monitored, especially in patients with pre-existing conditions or risk factors for the above conditions. Regular medical examinations, including blood tests and functional tests of the affected organ systems, are crucial to recognise potential adverse effects early and adjust treatment accordingly.

A holistic view of patient health and regular consideration of the risk-benefit ratio of therapy is essential to ensure that the benefits of weight loss outweigh the potential long-term risks. In some cases, this may mean considering alternative therapies or adjusting the dosage to minimise the risk of long-term health damage.

Risks for certain organ systems

The use of GLP-1 receptor agonists can put additional stress on the kidneys in people with pre-existing **renal impairment,** as these drugs can have both direct and indirect effects on kidney function.

Indirect effects include dehydration caused by side effects such as nausea and vomiting. These symptoms are particularly common at the beginning of therapy and can put a strain on the kidneys as they have less fluid available for the necessary filtration processes. The direct effects of the drugs on kidney function are not yet fully understood, but it is thought that they may affect the way blood flows through the kidneys and is filtered.

With long-term use of these drugs, there is concern that the cumulative effects could lead to a progressive deterioration of kidney function, especially in patients who already suffer from impaired kidney function. This can increase the risk of serious conditions such as chronic kidney disease or even kidney failure. For this reason, it is crucial to monitor kidney function regularly. This includes blood tests to determine serum creatinine and glomerular filtration rate, which are important indicators of kidney performance. Additional urine analyses can also be performed to detect early signs of kidney damage, such as the presence of protein in the urine.

If there are signs of deterioration in kidney function, it may be necessary to adjust the dosage of the medication or even consider an alternative treatment. Such decisions should be made in close co-operation with a doctor to ensure the safety and efficacy of the treatment and to protect the patient's health and quality of life.

Concerns about the risk of chronic or recurrent **pancreatitis with the** use of GLP-1 receptor agonists are also particularly relevant for patients who have a history of this condition. These drugs, which are commonly used to treat type 2 diabetes and aid weight loss, work by stimulating the GLP-1 receptor, which causes various physiological responses in the body, including influencing the secretion of digestive enzymes.

Stimulation of the GLP-1 receptor can cause increased secretion of digestive enzymes from the pancreas before food reaches the gut, which can lead to premature activation of these enzymes. Normally, these enzymes only become active in the intestine, where they can safely work to digest food. However, if they are activated too early, they can attack the pancreatic tissue instead, leading to inflammation. This mechanism could increase the risk of developing or worsening pancreatitis in patients using GLP-1 receptor agonists.

The treatment and management of patients who are susceptible to pancreatitis and use GLP-1 receptor agonists therefore require particularly careful monitoring. Symptoms of pancreatitis include severe abdominal pain that may radiate to the back, nausea, vomiting, fever and rapid heart rate. If these symptoms occur, patients should seek medical help immediately.

In addition, the healthcare provider should carefully consider the risks and benefits of continuing therapy with GLP-1 receptor agonists. In some cases, it may be necessary to adjust treatment or choose alternative therapeutic approaches to minimise the risk of pancreatitis. These decisions should be made on an individual basis, taking into account the patient's full medical history and personal circumstances to ensure safe and effective treatment.

Long-term hormonal and cellular effects

The long-term use of GLP-1 receptor agonists and their impact on hormonal balance is an important consideration for treatment, particularly in chronic conditions such as type 2 diabetes and obesity.

These drugs not only regulate blood glucose levels by influencing insulin secretion and delaying gastric emptying, but also have an effect on various hormones involved in the regulation of glucose metabolism.

GLP-1 receptor agonists stimulate the secretion of insulin, a key hormone that helps regulate blood sugar levels after a meal by promoting the uptake of glucose by cells. At the same time, these drugs suppress the release of glucagon, a hormone produced by the pancreas to increase blood sugar by promoting the release of stored sugar from the liver. By lowering glucagon secretion, GLP-1 receptor agonists help to reduce hepatic glucose production, which further lowers blood glucose levels.

These changes in insulin and glucagon balance can lead to effective control of blood glucose levels, but the long-term effects of these hormonal changes are not yet fully understood. There is a possibility that chronic interference with these hormones may affect other metabolic pathways, such as lipid metabolism or energy homeostasis, which could potentially lead to adverse effects.

These drugs could also have an influence on body weight by increasing the feeling of satiety and thus contributing to weight loss. This effect is largely positive, but persistent manipulation of satiety hormones and energy metabolism could disrupt the natural balance of hunger and satiety in the long term.

Given these potential effects, it is important that clinicians and patients carefully monitor the hormonal effects of GLP-1 receptor agonists and perform regular assessments to recognise and manage any potential adverse metabolic effects at an early stage. The decision to continue this therapy should always take into account the individual patient's response and include a continuous assessment of the risk-benefit ratio to ensure the patient's optimal long-term health and well-being.

The long-term stimulation of the GLP-1 receptor by certain diabetes and weight management drugs could also, according to some studies, influence cell growth and potentially increase the risk of certain types of cancer, including medullary thyroid carcinoma. These findings are mainly based on animal studies, which makes it difficult to interpret and transfer the results to humans.

Animal studies have also shown that activation of the GLP-1 receptor not only influences metabolic processes, but also promotes the growth and differentiation of certain cell types. Some studies have shown an increased rate of C-cell hyperplasia and tumours in rodents, particularly in the thyroid gland. C-cells are responsible for the production of calcitonin, and their hyperactivity can lead to medullary thyroid carcinoma, a rare but often aggressive type of cancer.

The relevance of these findings for humans remains controversial. While these animal-based data indicate a potential increase in risk, comparable effects in clinical use in humans have not been clearly demonstrated. Nevertheless, such results lead to increased caution and closer monitoring of patients treated with GLP-1 receptor agonists, especially those with a family history of medullary thyroid carcinoma or genetic diseases such as multiple endocrine neoplasia type 2, who are already at increased risk of such cancers.

Given these potential risks, it is recommended that patients using GLP-1 receptor agonists should have regular thyroid examinations to detect early signs of C-cell hyperplasia or other abnormal changes. At the same time, continued scientific research is needed to understand the mechanisms by which these drugs affect cell growth and to determine how great the risk to humans actually is. This knowledge is critical to ensure the safety of GLP-1 receptor agonist therapy and to make informed therapeutic decisions that balance long-term benefits against potential risks.

Contraindications

The use of weight loss injections, especially those containing GLP-1 receptor agonists, is contraindicated in certain patient groups due to the increased risk of serious side effects or complications. Important contraindications include:

- Medullary thyroid carcinoma and multiple endocrine neoplasia type 2 (MEN 2): People with a personal or family history of these diseases should avoid GLP-1 receptor agonists. Medullary thyroid carcinoma is a rare form of thyroid cancer that arises from the C-cells of the thyroid gland. MEN 2 is a genetic disorder that leads to various forms of endocrine neoplasia, including medullary thyroid carcinoma. The use of GLP-1 receptor agonists may increase the risk of developing these cancers due to the potential stimulatory effect on C-cell growth.

- Severe renal insufficiency: Patients with severe renal insufficiency or kidney disease should also be cautious or avoid GLP-1 receptor agonists. As previously mentioned, these drugs can place additional stress on kidney function, especially if kidney impairment is already present. Impaired renal function can impair the excretion of the drug and lead to accumulation, which increases the risk of side effects.
- Pancreatitis: Patients who suffer from pancreatitis or have a history of this condition should refrain from using GLP-1 receptor agonists. The drugs can increase the risk of recurrence of pancreatitis or worsening of the condition as they can affect the secretion of digestive enzymes, which can lead to inflammation.
- Gastrointestinal diseases: Patients with severe gastrointestinal conditions should use GLP-1 receptor agonists with caution. As these drugs can often cause side effects such as nausea, vomiting, diarrhoea and constipation, they can exacerbate existing conditions such as irritable bowel syndrome, ulcerative colitis or Crohn's disease.
- Pregnancy and lactation: There are insufficient data on the safety of GLP-1 receptor agonists during pregnancy and lactation. As a precaution, these drugs should be avoided during these

periods unless the benefit clearly outweighs the risk to the unborn child or infant.
- Cardiovascular disease: Although GLP-1 receptor agonists may have some beneficial effects on the cardiovascular system, individuals with severe cardiovascular disease such as advanced heart failure or unstable angina should consider using these medications only under close medical supervision.
- Severe liver disease: Individuals with severe liver disease should also exercise caution or avoid the use of GLP-1 receptor agonists. The liver plays a central role in the metabolism of many medications, and impaired liver function can affect the processing of these agents, leading to increased concentrations in the body and potentially toxic effects.
- Severe allergic reactions: Patients who have had severe allergic reactions to GLP-1 receptor agonist components in the past should not use this medication. Allergic reactions can range from skin rashes to anaphylaxis, a potentially life-threatening reaction.
- Alcohol abuse: Individuals who currently abuse alcohol or have a history of alcohol abuse should also be cautious, as alcohol can stress the pancreas and further increase the risk of pancreatitis. GLP-1 receptor agonists can further increase this risk.

For patients suffering from any of the above conditions, it is important to consider alternative treatments and work closely with healthcare providers to develop a safe and effective treatment plan. These precautions will help minimise the risk of serious complications and protect patients' health.

Precautionary measures

When using GLP-1 receptor agonists, it is essential to take special precautions, especially for people who already suffer from chronic diseases. These medications can potentially exacerbate existing health problems. Therefore, comprehensive and regular monitoring by healthcare professionals is crucial to ensure the safety and effectiveness of treatment.

Regular monitoring should include the following aspects:

- Blood tests: These are essential to monitor changes in blood glucose levels, kidney function, liver function and other important parameters that could be affected by the medication. Blood tests also help to assess the effectiveness of the treatment and to recognise early signs of complications.
- Monitoring renal function: As GLP-1 receptor agonists can lead to further damage in patients with renal insufficiency, it is particularly important to check renal function regularly. Tests

such as the measurement of serum creatinine and the calculation of the glomerular filtration rate (GFR) are standard.
- Dosage adjustments: Depending on the individual reactions to the therapy and the results of the regular checks, it may be necessary to adjust the dosage. This is particularly important for patients who show signs of side effects or in whom kidney or liver function deteriorates.

In addition, patients should be informed about possible side effects and symptoms that could indicate serious complications. These include gastrointestinal complaints, changes in urine, unexplained weight loss, yellowing of the skin or eyes, and severe abdominal pain. Such symptoms require immediate medical evaluation.

Close co-operation between patients and healthcare providers is important to ensure the safe use of GLP-1 receptor agonists. Patients should be encouraged to attend all medical appointments and report any changes in their health status without delay. This proactive approach will help to minimise potential risks and maximise the therapeutic benefits of this treatment.

Mixture of different medications

Combining or mixing different weight loss medications in the form of injections should be handled with caution and is not recommended without the express guidance and supervision of a qualified healthcare provider.

Different agents used for weight loss have specific mechanisms and modes of action, and combining them may result in unforeseen interactions, side effects or health risks.

- Pharmacological interactions: Different weight loss medications, such as GLP-1 receptor agonists (e.g. liraglutide, semaglutide), have different pharmacological properties. The combination of these drugs can lead to an increase or decrease in the effect of one or both drugs or even to new side effects.
- Increased side effects: Some of the most common side effects of GLP-1 agonists include nausea, vomiting, diarrhoea and possible irritation at the injection site. The combination of several of these drugs could increase the risk and severity of these side effects.
- Regulatory and clinical guidelines: To date, there is little clinical data on the safety and efficacy of combining different injectables for weight loss. Drugs are generally approved for use based on clinical trials that demonstrate their safety and efficacy as monotherapy or in a specific combination therapy.

Any type of combination therapy should only be used under the supervision and with the authorisation of a healthcare provider. It is important that patients inform their physicians of all medications they are taking, including those used for weight loss.

Which slimming injection for whom?

As shown, there are various types of medication on the market that differ in their mode of action and areas of application. The selection of a suitable medication depends on several factors, including individual health history, the presence of concomitant diseases, tolerability and the recommendations of the attending physician.

Selection by preparation

Here are some of the common types of weight loss injections and their typical applications:

GLP-1 receptor agonists (Wegovy, Saxenda, Trulicity)

The class of GLP-1 receptor agonists (glucagon-like peptide-1 agonists) is particularly effective for the treatment of overweight and obesity, especially in people with type 2 diabetes or prediabetes. The best-known drugs in this class include liraglutide (Saxenda), semaglutide (Wegovy) and dulaglutide (Trulicity). These drugs utilise an innovative approach to weight control and blood glucose regulation by mimicking and modulating the body's own mechanisms.

GLP-1 receptor agonists mimic the action of the natural hormone GLP-1, which is produced in the gut and plays a role in the regulation of blood glucose levels and appetite. The main effects of these drugs include

Increase in insulin secretion

GLP-1 receptor agonists utilise the hormone glucagon-like peptide-1, which is produced in the intestine and plays a central role in the regulation of blood sugar levels. When food is ingested and blood sugar rises, GLP-1 binds to receptors on the beta cells in the pancreas. This binding causes the beta cells to release more insulin, a hormone that is necessary to transport glucose from the blood into the cells. This leads to a drop in blood glucose levels. At the same time, GLP-1 helps to suppress the production of glucagon, a hormone produced by the alpha cells of the pancreas that increases blood glucose levels by stimulating the liver to release stored glucose. Reducing glucagon helps to keep blood sugar levels stable after a meal.

This dual mode of action of GLP-1 is particularly beneficial in the treatment of type 2 diabetes, as it helps to regulate blood glucose levels more effectively while reducing the likelihood of blood glucose peaks and troughs. As GLP-1 receptor agonists increase insulin secretion in a glucose-dependent manner, insulin secretion is only increased when blood glucose is high, but not when blood glucose is low, reducing the risk of hypoglycaemia. In addition to improving glycaemic control, these drugs also offer the benefit of weight loss by increasing satiety and delaying gastric emptying, ultimately leading to lower calorie intake. These properties make GLP-1 receptor agonists an effective treatment option that not only improves blood glucose levels, but also contributes to overall health improvement by assisting with weight management.

Reduction in the release of glucagon

GLP-1 receptor agonists not only influence insulin production, but also the amount of the hormone glucagon, which is secreted by the pancreas. Normally, glucagon helps to raise blood glucose levels by stimulating the liver to release stored glucose into the bloodstream. By reducing glucagon production, these drugs can lower blood sugar levels more effectively. This reduction is critical because it helps to mitigate meal-induced blood sugar spikes and thus improve blood sugar stability throughout the day.

This is particularly important for the treatment of type 2 diabetes, where consistent blood glucose control is crucial to avoid long-term health complications.

Delay in gastric emptying

GLP-1 receptor agonists affect the rate at which food leaves the stomach by slowing gastric emptying. This effect has benefits for weight control and the management of type 2 diabetes. When food stays in the stomach longer, this leads to a prolonged feeling of fullness. This prolonged feeling of fullness can help people eat less frequently or eat smaller portions because the urge to eat is dampened by the feeling of fullness.

The slower emptying of the stomach also plays an important role in blood sugar regulation. As food enters the small intestine more slowly, glucose is released into the blood more gradually, resulting in a more even and less spiky blood sugar curve after meals. This helps to reduce the typical post-meal blood sugar spikes that are common in people with diabetes and can lead to long-term health problems.

In addition, the slower gastric emptying induced by GLP-1 receptor agonists effectively supports weight management. By increasing and prolonging the feeling of satiety, these drugs help people to consume fewer calories, which can promote weight loss. This mechanism is particularly valuable as overweight and obesity are closely linked to the development and worsening of type 2 diabetes. The ability of these drugs to positively influence both glycaemic control and body weight makes them an important option in the treatment strategy for obese patients with type 2 diabetes.

Appetite regulation

GLP-1 receptor agonists have an interesting effect that goes beyond the direct effects on the stomach and pancreas. These drugs also affect the brain, leading to improved regulation of appetite and satiety. They do this by acting on specific areas of the brain that are responsible for regulating hunger and food intake. By activating these areas of the brain, the feeling of satiety is increased and appetite is reduced, causing patients to eat less.

The ability of these drugs to directly interfere with the central nervous system and amplify signals of well-being and fullness is crucial to their success in supporting weight loss. This process leads to a reduction in calorie intake because the prolonged feeling of fullness makes it easier to eat smaller meals and reduce snacking. This reduction in calorie intake is a natural consequence of feeling less hungry.

In addition, the effect of GLP-1 receptor agonists on the brain helps patients to change their eating habits and make healthier choices, which can lead to more sustainable weight management in the long term. This change in behaviour is particularly valuable as it helps to break the often difficult cycle of dieting and weight gain that plagues many people with obesity.

Overall, GLP-1 receptor agonists enable patients to control their calorie intake and achieve long-term weight loss through a combination of physical and psychological effects. This holistic approach to the treatment of obesity and type 2 diabetes makes them a valuable option in modern medical therapy.

Clinical application and benefits

For individuals with type 2 diabetes or prediabetes, these medications provide a dual function by helping to both reduce weight and improve glycaemic control. Weight management is an essential part of the treatment of type 2 diabetes, as overweight and obesity can exacerbate insulin resistance, which further exacerbates the disease.

The most common side effects of GLP-1 receptor agonists are gastrointestinal complaints such as nausea, vomiting, diarrhoea and constipation. These side effects are usually mild to moderate and often improve with time. There are also rare but more serious risks such as pancreatitis, kidney problems and possible thyroid tumours that need to be considered before starting treatment.

Amylin analogues (Symlin)

Amylin analogues, such as pramlintide (Symlin), represent a special class of diabetes drugs that are used to supplement insulin therapy. Pramlintide is a synthetic analogue of the human hormone amylin, which is naturally produced by the beta cells of the pancreas together with insulin. In people with diabetes, especially type 1 diabetes and type 2 diabetes, who use insulin, the production or effect of amylin is often insufficient.

Pramlintide works by mimicking the natural functions of amylin, which has several important effects on blood sugar control and food intake. Firstly, it slows the emptying of the stomach after a meal, resulting in a slower release of glucose into the bloodstream and thus reducing post-meal spikes in blood glucose levels. This slower gastric emptying also helps to prolong the feeling of fullness, which can reduce the total amount of food consumed. In addition, pramlintide inhibits the secretion of glucagon, a hormone that increases blood sugar levels by stimulating the liver to release glucose. By reducing glucagon secretion, pramlintide helps to further stabilise postprandial blood glucose levels.

Pramlintide is particularly suitable for patients with diabetes who cannot optimally control their blood glucose levels despite insulin therapy. It is of particular interest to type 1 diabetics who need additional control over blood glucose spikes and to type 2 diabetics who use insulin and have difficulty achieving their blood glucose targets. In addition, pramlintide may be of benefit to patients who are overweight or obese and also have diabetes, as it increases the feeling of satiety and can thus potentially contribute to weight loss.

Pramlintide offers valuable support for patients on structured diabetes therapy who are constantly struggling with fluctuations in blood glucose levels. It helps to moderate glucose uptake after meals, making it easier to achieve and maintain more stable blood glucose levels. The use of pramlintide requires careful coordination and monitoring by a doctor, as the dosage of insulin may need to be adjusted to avoid hypoglycaemia.

Overall, pramlintide improves patients' quality of life through better glycaemic control and supports weight management goals, making it an important adjunct in the treatment of diabetes, especially for those already using insulin.

Combination preparations (Contrave)

Bupropion/naltrexone, known under the trade name Contrave, is a weight loss medication that combines two active ingredients that work synergistically to influence appetite and hunger. This drug is particularly interesting because it intervenes in a unique way in the neurochemical processes of the brain that affect eating behaviour as well as moods and possible addiction mechanisms.

Bupropion is an active ingredient that was originally used as an antidepressant and for smoking cessation. It acts primarily as a dopamine and noradrenaline reuptake inhibitor, which means that it increases the availability of these neurotransmitters in the brain. Dopamine plays a central role in reward and motivation and can also influence food cravings, particularly for sweet or fatty foods, which are often associated with reward signalling. Noradrenaline, on the other hand, is involved in the regulation of alertness and energy expenditure.

Naltrexone, the second drug in the combination, is normally used to treat alcohol and opiate addiction. It acts as an opioid receptor antagonist, which means that it blocks the effects of opioids that occur naturally in the brain and are part of the body's reward system. By blocking these receptors, naltrexone can help to reduce the cravings and reward sensations associated with eating.

The combination of bupropion and naltrexone in Contrave utilises these mechanisms to reduce appetite and increase satiety. By improving mood and providing increased alertness, while naltrexone curbs the rewarding aspects of eating, the overall desire for food is reduced. This makes Contrave an effective option for individuals struggling with overweight or obesity, especially when these conditions are associated with emotional aspects such as stress eating or low mood.

In addition to weight loss, Contrave may also be suitable for people who are also struggling with addictive behaviour or mood disorders. The antidepressant properties of bupropion can be supportive for patients with depressive disorders, and the addiction-suppressing properties of naltrexone can be helpful when eating behaviour is seen as part of an addiction problem.

The drug is usually used as part of a comprehensive weight management treatment plan that includes dietary changes, physical activity and behavioural changes. Before using Contrave, it is important to seek medical advice as the drug may interact with other medications and is not suitable for every patient. It can cause side effects such as nausea, constipation, headaches and occasionally increased blood pressure, which need to be monitored and assessed by a doctor.

Health status as a selection criterion

When selecting a weight loss injection, as used in the treatment of overweight and obesity, numerous factors must be considered to ensure that the medication is effective and safe. The patient's state of health plays a central role in this.

Existing conditions such as diabetes can significantly influence the choice of medication. For example, GLP-1 receptor agonists may be particularly suitable in such cases, as they not only help with weight management but also improve blood glucose control. These drugs can therefore be doubly beneficial for diabetics who want to lose weight.

Cardiovascular diseases are also important when choosing a weight loss medication. Some medications can affect the cardiovascular system, for example by increasing blood pressure or heart rate. Here it is important to choose a medication that is safe for patients with such pre-existing conditions or to adjust the dosage accordingly.

Mental health problems such as depression or anxiety disorders must also be taken into account, as some weight loss medications can have an impact on mood and well-being. Medications that affect the central nervous system, such as bupropion, which also has antidepressant effects, may be favoured in such cases.

Choosing the right medication for weight loss must therefore always be an individualised decision based on a comprehensive medical assessment. It is important that doctors consider all aspects of the patient's health to ensure safe and effective treatment. Possible interactions with other medications the patient may be taking, as well as individual circumstances and needs, should also be factored into the decision-making process.

Interactions with other medications as a criterion

Checking for interactions between a weight loss injection and other medications a patient may be taking is another critical step in the safe and effective treatment of overweight or obesity. Drug interactions can reduce the effectiveness of treatment, increase unwanted side effects or even cause dangerous health problems.

For example, GLP-1 receptor agonists, which are commonly used for weight loss, can have potential interactions with a variety of other medications. They can affect the rate at which drugs are released from the stomach, which can alter the absorption and effectiveness of these drugs. This is particularly relevant for medications that require precise dosing, such as oral antidiabetics or blood pressure medications.

When using bupropion/naltrexone, another common option for weight loss injections, doctors need to be aware of the combination with other substances with a central nervous system effect, such as certain antidepressants or antipsychotics. Bupropion can increase the risk of seizures, especially in combination with drugs that lower the seizure threshold.

It is also important to consider the interaction between weight loss injections and medications that affect the risk of bleeding, as some of these weight loss medications can affect blood clotting. This could lead to complications in patients taking anticoagulants such as warfarin.

Assessing such interactions requires careful consideration and sometimes adjustment of the dosage or schedule of medication use. It is imperative that physicians and pharmacists review a complete list of all medications, including prescription, over-the-counter and herbal products, that a patient is using before prescribing a weight loss injection. Patients should also be encouraged to report any changes to their medication or new medications started to ensure that their treatment plan remains safe and effective.

Side effects as a selection criterion

When choosing weight loss injections, the potential side effects must also be carefully considered, as these can affect the patient's quality of life and sometimes pose serious health risks. The most common side effects associated with these medications, such as nausea, vomiting, diarrhoea and constipation, are often an expression of the drug's effect on the gastrointestinal tract. These symptoms may occur particularly during the initial phase of treatment and may diminish over time as the body becomes accustomed to the medication.

The slowing of gastric emptying, a common effect of many weight loss medications, can lead to nausea and constipation. While this effect can contribute to weight loss by prolonging the feeling of fullness, the associated discomfort can be difficult to manage for some patients. Diarrhoea and vomiting can also occur as the body reacts to the change in food intake and the active ingredients in the medication.

In addition, there are more serious but less common side effects that need to be considered when deciding on a particular weight loss injection. For example, the risk of pancreatitis, an inflammation of the pancreas, may be increased with the use of some GLP-1 receptor agonists. This is a serious medical condition that requires immediate treatment. Kidney problems can also occur, especially if the medication impairs fluid absorption or if there is already pre-existing kidney damage.

Choosing the right medication should therefore not only be based on efficacy, but also take into account the patient's individual tolerance and risk profile. It is important that doctors and patients work together to weigh up the pros and cons of each treatment option, including considering how side effects might affect the patient's day-to-day lifestyle and general health. Open communication about any side effects experienced and a willingness to adjust treatment if necessary are crucial to ensure that treatment is not only effective but also safe.

Long-term effects as a selection criterion

Choosing a weight loss injection as part of a comprehensive weight management plan that includes dietary changes, physical activity and behavioural therapy is an important step in achieving long-term weight loss success. In fact, the suitability of different types of weight loss injections for long-term treatment varies depending on their mode of action, effectiveness, safety profile and patient tolerance.

Some of the more commonly used weight loss injections are based on GLP-1 receptor agonists, such as liraglutide, semaglutide and dulaglutide. These drugs are not only effective in reducing body weight, but also have positive effects on glucose metabolism, which makes them particularly useful for patients with type 2 diabetes. Their effect on slowing gastric emptying and improving insulin secretion makes them an attractive option for long-term therapy, especially because they can also reduce the risk of cardiovascular disease.

These medications are generally well suited for long-term use as they help to improve overall metabolic health in addition to weight loss. Patients using GLP-1 receptor agonists often report a sustained improvement in satiety and a reduction in calorie intake, making it easier to maintain the reduced body weight.

The tolerability and safety profile of the drugs are also crucial for the decision to use them in long-term therapy. GLP-1 receptor agonists are generally well tolerated, although they can cause side effects such as nausea and indigestion in some patients. These side effects are often temporary and can be alleviated by adjusting the dosage or other supportive measures.

In addition to GLP-1 receptor agonists, there are other classes of medication such as the combination of bupropion and naltrexone that may also be suitable for long-term use, particularly in patients who are also struggling with psychological factors such as depression or addictive behaviour. These medications can help address the emotional aspect of eating behaviour, which for some patients can be a key factor in the fight against obesity.

The choice of the right slimming injection for long-term treatment therefore depends on individual factors such as the patient's state of health, concomitant illnesses, the safety profile of the medication and the patient's individual response to the treatment.

Availability as a selection criterion

The availability of weight loss injections can also be an important selection criterion for people considering weight loss medication. Due to the growing popularity of this treatment method and certain production limitations, there may be regional shortages. This shortage can have various causes:

- Production capacities: The production of drug delivery syringes can be complex and place specific demands on the production environment and technology. If these capacities are limited, this can lead to supply bottlenecks.
- Regulatory authorisations: In some countries or regions, regulatory hurdles can affect the availability of these drugs. The authorisation procedures can be lengthy, which delays the market launch of new products.
- Surplus demand: In the event of a sudden increase in demand, for example due to positive study results or public interest, the existing production capacity may not be sufficient to meet demand.
- Distribution and logistics problems: Global or local logistics problems, such as those caused by political changes or pandemics, also influence the availability of such medicines.

It is therefore advisable for people considering treatment with weight loss injections to find out about the availability in their region at an early stage and possibly consider alternatives if these drugs are difficult to obtain. It is also important to view treatment in a comprehensive context that includes diet and exercise to achieve the best results and not be solely dependent on the availability of a single medication.

Costs as a selection criterion

The cost of weight loss injections is another key selection criterion for many people considering weight loss medication. The financial aspects can significantly influence the accessibility and decision for or against such treatment.

Market prices and manufacturers

The cost of weight loss injections can vary depending on the manufacturer and country. Patented drugs are often more expensive than their generic counterparts. The price can also be influenced by factors such as market exclusivity, production costs and the manufacturer's pricing policy.

The cost of weight loss injections varies depending on the specific medication, dosage and the country's healthcare system.

On average, the cost of Wegovy, which is used for weight loss at higher doses, can be around 200 to 300 euros/USD per month, depending on the pharmacy and dosage requirements. Saxenda can cost slightly less, but is often in the 200 Euro/USD per month range. These prices can vary depending on the individual dosage and the number of syringes required each month.

Additional costs

In addition to the direct costs of the injections themselves, additional expenses for regular medical examinations, consultations and possible side-effect treatments may also have to be taken into account.

Insurance cover

The issue of health insurance coverage for weight loss medication is a difficult and inconsistently treated topic that is strongly influenced by national healthcare systems and specific insurance policies.

In many countries, certain criteria such as a defined BMI index must be met for the costs to be covered by health insurance. Typically, such treatments are only covered by insurance if other, less invasive methods of weight loss, such as diet and exercise, have previously been tried and have been unsuccessful. The practice is often inconsistent within a country and is also volatile because the practice of weight loss injections, which are still relatively new, is not yet established.

Accompanying medical conditions also play a significant role. Individuals who suffer from disease-related weight problems, such as type 2 diabetes or high blood pressure, are often more likely to qualify for coverage of drug treatments, as these may be considered necessary for the treatment of the underlying conditions. In these cases, doctors and patients argue that weight reduction not only benefits quality of life, but can also reduce overall costs to the healthcare system by reducing other health complications.

However, the specific policies and the resulting decisions of health insurers vary considerably. In some countries, healthcare systems are more orientated towards supporting preventative measures and may therefore be more inclined to cover such treatments. In other countries, however, coverage is less likely unless the patient fulfils a long list of requirements.

In Germany, for example, statutory health insurance companies do not generally cover the costs of GLP-1 receptor agonists for weight loss, such as Wegovy (semaglutide) or Saxenda (liraglutide), as a standard weight loss treatment. The main use of these drugs under health insurance coverage is focused on specific medical conditions that go beyond the mere desire for weight loss.

However, the assumption of costs may be considered if the following conditions are met:

- Presence of obesity: As a rule, the patient must have a body mass index (BMI) of at least 30 kg/m², which is considered obesity. In some cases, especially if there are additional health problems, costs can be covered even if the BMI is 27 kg/m².
- Additional health complications: Patients with diabetes-related complications or other weight-related health problems such as high blood

pressure, sleep apnoea or certain cardiovascular diseases could also be eligible for coverage.
- Failure of conventional measures: Usually, conventional methods of weight loss, such as diet and exercise, must have been tried and judged unsuccessful. A medically supervised weight management programme that has not shown sufficient results could also be a criterion.

It is important that the treating doctor provides detailed medical justification and documentation for the necessity of this treatment, as health insurance companies often refuse to cover the costs without this. The decision can also vary from health insurance company to health insurance company, and it is advisable to discuss the possibilities and conditions of cost coverage directly with your own health insurance company.

The coverage decision is also often influenced by economic considerations. The cost of drug treatments for weight loss can be high, and insurers must weigh the potential long-term savings from reduced health problems against the immediate cost of medication.

It is therefore advisable for patients who are considering such treatment to find out exactly what their health insurance covers and, if necessary, to speak to medical professionals about the possibilities of having these costs reimbursed.

Optimal use of weight loss syringes

To maximise the effectiveness of weight loss injections while minimising risks and side effects, it is important to take a comprehensive approach that includes correct use and dosage, combination with diet plans and exercise programmes, and regular monitoring and adjustment of treatment.

Correct application and dosage

The use of weight loss injections, especially GLP-1 receptor agonists, requires careful patient guidance and training to ensure effective and safe use. The process begins with thorough education on the correct handling and administration of the medication.

Training for self-injection

Patients who use weight loss syringes must be instructed in the technique of self-injection. This includes the correct drawing up of the medication from the vial or the handling of pre-filled pens. Training should also include a demonstration of how to remove the protective cap, fit the needle securely and prepare the syringe for injection. It is important that patients learn how to remove air bubbles from the syringe to ensure accurate dosing.

Selection of the injection site

Subcutaneous injection allows the medication to be administered directly under the skin, which promotes slow and even absorption of the active ingredient. Typical injection sites include the abdomen, thigh and upper arm. These areas are favoured because they are easily accessible and provide sufficient subcutaneous fatty tissue, making the injection less painful. Patients should be instructed to change injection sites with each application to minimise the risk of skin irritation, lipodystrophy or infection. Systematically changing sites can help to keep the tissue healthy and optimise the absorption of the drug.

Dosing instructions

The dosage of slimming injections must be individually adjusted to achieve maximum efficacy with minimised side effects. The initial dosage is often low and is gradually increased based on the patient's tolerance and reactions. This gradual increase helps the body to become accustomed to the medication and can reduce the frequency and severity of side effects such as nausea and vomiting. The exact dosage and schedule for the increase should be clearly communicated to ensure that the patient follows the guidelines exactly.

Monitoring and customisation

Continuous monitoring by healthcare professionals is crucial to assess the patient's response to treatment and adjust the dosage accordingly. Regular follow-up visits allow the doctor to assess the effectiveness of the treatment and respond to possible side effects. These appointments also provide an opportunity to review and correct the self-injection technique, which is particularly important to ensure the patient's long-term adherence and well-being.

By implementing these comprehensive education and monitoring strategies, patients can not only improve their ability to self-manage their treatment, but also increase their chances of successful and sustainable weight loss.

Combination with nutrition plans and exercise programmes

Weight loss injections can contribute significantly to weight loss, especially when used as part of a comprehensive weight management programme that includes carefully tailored diet and exercise plans. This integrative approach recognises that sustainable weight loss and health promotion cannot be achieved through medication alone, but requires a comprehensive lifestyle change.

Nutrition plans

A well thought out nutritional strategy is crucial to maximise the effect of weight loss injections. A nutrient-rich, calorie-controlled diet not only helps achieve the calorie deficit necessary for weight loss, but also helps the body obtain all the necessary vitamins, minerals and other nutrients required for optimal health. Such diet plans should include the following aspects:

- Balanced macronutrient distribution: Carbohydrates, proteins and fats should be in a ratio that meets individual needs, for example, more proteins for satiety and muscle building support and healthy fats that provide long-term energy and promote heart health.
- Include whole foods: Fruits, vegetables, whole grains and lean proteins are essential because they provide fewer calories with higher nutritional value, helping to control hunger and cravings.
- Limit processed foods and sugar: These can disrupt insulin levels and lead to weight gain. Reducing them can not only help with weight control, but also reduce the risk of diabetes and other metabolic diseases.

Exercise programmes

Physical activity is another central pillar in the treatment of obesity and should include both aerobic exercise and strength training:

- Aerobic exercise: Activities such as running, swimming or cycling improve cardiovascular health and burn calories, which directly contributes to weight loss. Regular aerobic exercise also improves insulin sensitivity, which is particularly important for people with or on the verge of diabetes.
- Strength training: Building muscle mass is crucial, as muscles burn more calories than fatty tissue, even at rest. Strength training not only strengthens muscles, but also improves bone density and general body composition.

Regular review and adjustment

Combining these elements into a comprehensive plan requires careful monitoring and regular adjustments to ensure that goals are met and health is maintained. This means regular meetings with a nutritionist and a fitness trainer, as well as ongoing medical monitoring by the doctor prescribing the weight loss injections. Adjustments may be necessary in response to changes in lifestyle, health conditions or simply the body's response to previous treatment.

By taking these aspects into account, weight management with weight loss injections not only becomes more effective, but also more sustainable by helping patients develop healthy habits that lead to better health in the long term.

Medical monitoring of the treatment

Regular medical monitoring is essential to ensure that treatment with weight loss injections remains safe and effective. This includes regular checks of weight, blood pressure, blood sugar levels and other relevant health indicators.

Treatment should be able to be adapted flexibly to respond to changes in the patient's response or the occurrence of side effects. Dosages can be adjusted, medication can be changed or additional support measures can be recommended, depending on individual needs.

In collaboration with nutritionists, physiotherapists and other healthcare professionals, regular adjustments can be made based on the latest medical findings and the patient's personal development. This interdisciplinary approach is crucial to ensure long-term success and improve the patient's quality of life.

Duration of treatment

Weight loss injections are often part of a long-term treatment strategy. These medications, which are often injected once a week, can help to reduce feelings of hunger and promote weight loss. However, it is precisely this long-term nature that leads to a challenge in terms of cost.

The long-term nature of this treatment means that the total cost includes not only the purchase of the medication, but also regular visits to the doctor to monitor progress and possible side effects. Over months or even years, these costs can be significant and represent a financial hurdle for many patients.

The assumption of costs by health insurers varies greatly. In countries with comprehensive healthcare systems or insurance policies that promote preventative treatments, these costs may be partially or fully covered. In other cases, patients may have to pay most or all of the costs themselves, which can limit the accessibility of this treatment.

It is also important to note that the effectiveness and need for continued use of these injections should be reviewed regularly. Not every patient will have the desired results from these treatments and it is possible that adjustments to treatment methods may be required, which may incur additional costs.

It can be helpful for those affected to discuss the expected costs and duration of treatment in detail with their doctor and health insurance provider. It may also be useful to ask about generic alternatives or seek support from government healthcare programmes or pharmaceutical manufacturers' patient assistance programmes, which in some cases offer financial support for long-term treatment.

Interruption of treatment

Treatment with weight loss injections containing GLP-1 receptor agonists such as semaglutide or liraglutide can theoretically be interrupted, but this should be done carefully and ideally in consultation with a doctor. There are various reasons why such treatment might be interrupted, but it is important to understand the possible consequences of interruption.

- Efficacy: GLP-1 receptor agonists work by regulating appetite and improving insulin sensitivity. They achieve their full effectiveness through continuous use. Discontinuation can lead to a loss of progress in weight management as the underlying mechanism of appetite control and improved metabolic activity is no longer maintained.
- Weight management: Many users experience weight regain after stopping medication, as the original physiological conditions that led to overweight or obesity often remain unchanged. Regaining weight can be discouraging and undermine long-term weight management goals.
- Medical supervision: If the decision is made to interrupt treatment, this should be done under medical supervision. The doctor can help to organise the interruption in such a way that

possible negative effects are minimised and can advise on how treatment can be safely resumed at a later date.
- Side effects and tolerability: In some cases, it may be advisable to interrupt treatment, particularly if side effects occur or health problems arise that make further use of the medication inadvisable. In such cases, an interruption may be necessary to protect the patient's health or to evaluate alternative treatment options.
- Cost and accessibility: The high cost and potentially limited availability of the medication can of course also be reasons for interruption, especially if they are not sustainable in the long term.

In all cases, it is advisable to make such a decision with a healthcare provider to ensure that it is in the best interest of the patient's health and long-term goals. Alternatives and support strategies should also be considered to ensure continuity of weight management.

Sources of supply

There are various ways to obtain weight loss injections:

- Medical prescription: In Europe, the USA and many other countries, weight loss injections require a prescription. This means that a doctor must determine the need for this treatment and issue a prescription. This is the usual way to ensure that the treatment is medically appropriate and safe for the patient.
- Specialists in endocrinology or diabetology: It is often specialists in endocrinology or diabetology who prescribe such medication, as they specialise in metabolic diseases and hormonal imbalances. These doctors can carry out a comprehensive health assessment and determine whether treatment with GLP-1 receptor agonists is suitable.
- Weight management clinics: Many healthcare facilities that specialise in weight management also offer access to drug treatments such as weight loss injections. These clinics often have teams of doctors, dietitians and other professionals who offer an integrated approach to weight loss. They also often offer financial plans for treatment.
- Online pharmacies and telemedicine: Some online pharmacies and telemedicine providers can also issue prescriptions for weight loss

injections after an online consultation with a qualified doctor. This can be a convenient option for patients who live in remote areas or have difficulty seeing a doctor in person. However, it is important to ensure that these services are licensed and regulated to avoid risks.
- Direct purchase at the pharmacy with a prescription: After receiving a prescription, the medication can be purchased at almost any pharmacy. Pharmacists can also provide additional information on the correct use and storage of the medication.

Ethical and social considerations

The ethical debate about weight loss injections raises a number of moral issues. This debate touches on issues such as body image standards, access to medical care and the question of how far medical interventions to alter natural body conditions should go. We will only touch on these issues here, as they are in fact becoming increasingly marginalised.

Weight loss injections offer valuable medical support for people for whom conventional methods such as diet and exercise alone are not sufficient to achieve a healthy weight. These medications are a particularly important option for people with obesity or excess weight that has already led to health complications such as type 2 diabetes or cardiovascular disease. Due to the effective weight reduction made possible by these injections, many of the people affected can experience an improvement in their health situation. This can lead to reduced dependence on other medications, promote better physical performance and improve overall quality of life.

In addition, weight loss injections help to raise awareness and understanding of obesity as a chronic condition. By addressing it medically, the stigma often associated with obesity can be reduced. This leads to greater empathy and support for those affected, helping them to feel less isolated and more socially accepted.

It is also important to recognise that the development of such medical treatments is the result of extensive research and innovation aimed at providing viable solutions to serious health problems. These advances in medicine strengthen people's right to self-determination over their health and enable personalised treatments that were previously not possible.

Overall, weight loss injections offer many people a life-changing improvement in their health and quality of life. They are an example of how medical innovation can help overcome the challenges of chronic illness and help those affected to lead a more active and healthy life.

In addition, weight loss injections offer an effective treatment option for people who suffer from unhealthy obesity and for whom other methods such as diet and exercise have not been successful. For these people, injections can not only enable weight loss but also lead to an improvement in associated health conditions such as type 2 diabetes, cardiovascular disease and others. It is often argued here that access to such treatments is a matter of medical justice and can help people live healthier and potentially longer lives.

The increasing normalisation of weight loss injections will help to reduce the stigmatisation of overweight and obesity by recognising them as treatable medical conditions. By recognising obesity as a condition that requires medical intervention, this could help to reduce blame and self-blame among those affected.

However, there are naturally also concerns about the ethics of medical interventions that aim to alter the body. Some see this as a rejection of the acceptance of natural body diversity. On the other hand, supporters argue that access to such treatments strengthens people's right to self-determination in making decisions about their bodies and health.

Overall, the discussion around weight loss injections is complex and raises important questions about our society's priorities, understanding of health and the role of medicine in our lives. It remains important that these discussions are held to ensure a balanced understanding of the pros and cons of such medical interventions.

According to the authors, however, the positive factors of weight loss injections clearly outweigh the negative ones.

New drugs, conclusion and outlook

Weight loss injections are already better than their reputation. For the first time, they have the potential to effectively combat the widespread disease of obesity. There is no need to emphasise what this can mean for those affected.

Further improvements in weight loss injections could be significant in the future. Researchers are working on increasing the effectiveness of these drugs by targeting the relevant metabolic pathways more effectively. The aim is to achieve stronger and longer-lasting effects on weight loss while minimising side effects. The development of new combination therapies that bring together different active ingredients to promote weight loss also shows promising approaches. These could improve the effectiveness of the treatment while reducing the dosages of the individual components, which increases tolerability.

Another significant advance could lie in the form of administration of these drugs. Currently, they are mostly administered as injections, but research could lead to more convenient forms such as oral doses or implantable devices that release the drug continuously. Research is also looking at personalised medicine approaches, where treatment is tailored specifically to patients' individual genetic, metabolic and physiological characteristics in order to optimise therapy.

The future role of **cortisol**, a hormone known to regulate metabolism and the body's response to stress, is also important. High cortisol levels can lead to weight gain and influence appetite and fat storage behaviour. Future therapies could aim to modulate cortisol levels or mitigate the effects of cortisol on the body to improve the effectiveness of weight loss injections. This could be done through combination therapies that not only contain GLP-1 agonists, but also components that specifically address the metabolic effects caused by cortisol.

Tirzepatide, a relatively new active ingredient in the treatment of type 2 diabetes, also shows promising results in the area of weight reduction and could play an important role in weight loss injections in the future. Tirzepatide is a dual agonist that activates both the glucagon-like peptide-1 (GLP-1) receptor and the glucose-dependent insulinotropic polypeptide (GIP) receptor. These properties make it particularly effective in both controlling blood glucose levels and reducing body weight.

In clinical trials, tirzepatide has shown very good results in terms of weight loss. For example, the phase 3 SURMOUNT-1 study showed that participants treated with tirzepatide achieved a very significant weight loss of up to 20% of their body weight. This exceeds the results achieved with current GLP-1 agonists such as semaglutide, which are also used for weight loss.

The mode of action of tirzepatide involves several mechanisms: it improves insulin sensitivity, slows gastric emptying and increases the feeling of satiety, which leads to reduced calorie intake. These effects are particularly beneficial for people who have difficulty reducing their weight through diet and exercise alone.

Based on these promising results, tirzepatide is expected to play an increasingly important role in the development of weight loss injections in the future. However, the approval and market launch of tirzepatide as a weight loss agent will still take some time, as the final phases of clinical trials and the approval process have to be completed.

The prospects for the further development and improvement of weight loss injections are therefore promising and focus on increased efficacy, ease of use and personalised treatment options that have the potential to further improve the quality of life for many people.

It is also expected that weight loss injections - like many new drugs - will become less expensive over time. The future of pricing for weight loss injections, such as GLP-1 receptor agonists, is dependent on several factors, but there are reasons for cautious optimism that they could become more affordable over time. As demand for these drugs increases, manufacturers could benefit from economies of scale that allow them to lower prices. In addition, technological advances and more efficient production methods could lead to a reduction in manufacturing costs. Another significant influencing factor is the expiry of patents for existing drugs, which paves the way for cheaper generics. Regulatory decisions and healthcare policies aimed at reducing the cost of medicines could also play a role. Although the pricing of medicines is complex and dependent on many variable market and political factors, these developments give us hope that the cost of prescription syringes will fall in the future.